The Complete Guidebook On The Causes, Symptom, Diagnosis, Treatment And Management

Dr. Albert Nicole

Table of Contents

CHAPTER ONE 3

    AFib 3

    What Kind Of Effects Does Having Atrial Fibrillation Have On My Body? 8

    The Typical Functioning Of Your Heart 9

CHAPTER TWO 17

    Who Is Susceptible To Developing Atrial Fibrillation 17

    Different Kinds Of Afib 18

    Is It Possible That Anxiety Could 22

CHAPTER THREE 24

    Diagnosis..24

    Treatment For Patients Suffering From Atrial Fibrillation (Afib) 28

THE END 52

CHAPTER ONE

AFib

Atrial fibrillation, also known as AF, is a form of arrhythmia, also known as an abnormal heartbeat. The abbreviation "afib" refers to this condition. Afib is brought on by abnormally rapid and erratic heartbeats that originate in the upper chambers of the heart (usually more than 400 beats per minute).

A regular contraction of the heart muscle is essential to the maintenance of a regular and healthy heartbeat. When at rest, a contraction occurs approximately once per second, but this frequency increases with exercise. The blood is pushed down into the ventricles from the atria, which are the two upper chambers of the heart, with each contraction (the two lower chambers). After that, the ventricles will contract, which will force the blood to either the lungs or the remainder of the body.

But in a person who has atrial fibrillation, the atria contract in an irregular manner and at a rate that is much higher than what is considered normal. After that, the atria are no longer beating in time with the ventricles. The atrium is a common location for blood pooling, which increases the risk of both blood clots and strokes. In some patients with atrial fibrillation, the condition known as atrial flutter can lead to heart failure.

Afib could happen once in a while, or it could be present all the time.

What symptoms do you experience when you have atrial fibrillation?

A single electrical impulse from the sinus node, which is a single point in the right atrium of the heart, triggers the beginning of a normal heartbeat. Heart rates typically range from 60 to 150 beats per minute in healthy individuals.

Electrical impulses can originate from a number of different locations within the patient's atria when they have Afib. Because of this, the atria may contract at a rate of more than 400 times per minute. When the ventricles try to keep up with the contractions, they become overworked and exhausted. They beat faster than they should, so there is a possibility that they do not have enough time to fill with blood and pump blood in the normal manner.

Because of this, blood tends to collect in the atria rather than flowing into the ventricles and then being distributed to the rest of the body. Because of this pooling, there is an increased risk of blood clots forming in the heart. Clots of blood can form in the heart, travel through the bloodstream, and then lodge themselves in the brain, which can result in a stroke.

What Kind Of Effects Does Having Atrial Fibrillation Have On My Body?

When you have atrial fibrillation (Afib), the electrical system in your heart isn't functioning as it should. Your electrical impulses are a mess, which is leading to your heart beating in an irregular and rapid pattern. When you notice something is off with your pulse, you might find yourself wondering what's going on in your heart. It is helpful to gain a better understanding of the differences that exist between a normal heartbeat and what occurs when you are experiencing Afib.

The Typical Functioning Of Your Heart

Your heart is the organ responsible for pumping blood to the rest of your body. Your two atriums are the first chambers to contract during each heartbeat, by your two lower (ventricles). When at precisely the right hese actions enable your ınction as an effective electrical system of your heart is responsible for controlling the timing of your heart's contractions. In most cases, the sinoatrial (SA) node is the one in charge of the electrical system in your body. This node can be found in the right atrium of your structure. Electrical activity spreads through your right and left atria ("atrium" is singular and "atria" is plural) whenever your SA node generates an impulse ("atrium" is singular and "atria" is plural). After that, both of your atriums will contract, which will cause blood to be forced into your ventricles.

After reaching it, the impulse moves on to the atrioventricular (AV) node, which is situated close to the center of your heart. After that, the impulse travels to your ventricles, which triggers the ventricles to contract and force blood to be pumped out of your heart and into your lungs as well as the rest of your body. This process occurs again and again with each beat of the heart. The SA node is responsible for directing the timing of the electrical impulses and ensuring that your heart continues to pump effectively.

You can compare the SA node in your network to the conductor of an orchestra. Your SA node is in charge of ensuring that your heart is beating at the appropriate rate and rhythm at all times. In a similar manner, the conductor of an orchestra directs all of the musicians to ensure that the music continues to flow at the appropriate tempo, which can vary from time to time from faster to slower.

In a normal situation, your SA node will adapt to the amount of activity you are doing. When you exercise, for instance, the rate of impulses increases, but when you sleep, the rate decreases. Another example is that it has the opposite effect when you sleep. Because the SA node is controlling the rhythm of your heart, you are said to be in "normal sinus rhythm." This indicates that your heart beats at a consistent rhythm and rate, which is somewhere between 60 and 100 times per minute.

What can you expect if you are diagnosed with Afib?

If you have atrial fibrillation, the SA node in your heart is not properly directing the electrical rhythm of your heart. Instead, a number of distinct impulses fire off in a frenzied manner at the same time, leading to a rapid and disorganized rhythm in your atrium. As a direct consequence of this, your atria are unable to effectively contract and pump blood into your ventricles. Because of this, your ventricles contract in an abnormal manner, which results in a rapid and irregular heartbeat.

It's as if two more conductors walked onto the stage in the middle of the performance and started waving their batons around. The musicians would have no idea who to follow or what to do once that information was lost.

Without rhythm and harmony, the music would be unlistenable.

If you suffer from atrial fibrillation (Afib), you are in luck because there are many ways to restore rhythm and harmony to your heart. It all begins with a visit to your primary care physician, who will conduct some diagnostic tests and make a determination about your condition.

How common is the condition known as atrial fibrillation?

Researchers have referred to atrial fibrillation (Afib) as the "new cardiovascular disease epidemic of the 21st century." Afib is particularly prevalent among people of advanced age. Over 33 million people worldwide aged 55 and older have been diagnosed with the condition. Afib is expected to affect 12 million people in the United States by the year 2030, according to estimates. Afib is responsible for almost half a million annual hospitalizations in the United States and contributes to an increasing number of fatalities with each passing year.

CHAPTER TWO

Who Is Susceptible To Developing Atrial Fibrillation

Although anyone can be diagnosed with atrial fibrillation, the condition is more prevalent in people of European descent. On the other hand, Black people who have atrial fibrillation have a significantly increased risk of experiencing serious complications, such as a stroke or heart failure. It is more common to diagnose individuals who were assigned the female gender at birth (AFAB) than individuals who were assigned the male gender at birth (AMAB).

Different Kinds Of Afib

There are three categories of atrial fibrillation, which are as follows:

• Paroxysmal Afib: This form of Afib is characterized by episodes of irregular heart rhythm that resolve on their own after a period of seven days.

• Persistent atrial fibrillation is a form of atrial fibrillation that continues for more than a week. In contrast to paroxysmal Afib, it may call for cardioversion, also known as giving the heart an electric shock, in order to return it to a normal rhythm.

- Long-standing persistent Afib: This condition is very similar to persistent Afib; however, it continues for more than a year.

What signs and symptoms are associated with atrial fibrillation?

There are times when atrial fibrillation does not cause any symptoms at all, and you might not even be aware that you have it. When it does cause symptoms, some of those symptoms may include the following:

- Angina (chest pain caused by a reduced blood supply to the heart muscle)

- Dizziness

- Fainting (also known as syncope); • Fatigue; • Palpitations (the sensation that one's heart is skipping beats or beating too quickly); • Weakness; • Shortness of Breath

Afib can also result in some serious complications, including the following:

- Thromboembolic disease • Congestive heart failure

- Stroke

What factors contribute to the development of atrial fibrillation?

Atrial fibrillation is a condition that is caused by alterations or damage to the tissue and electrical system of the heart. The majority of the time, coronary artery disease or high blood pressure are the culprits behind these changes. Atrial fibrillation is frequently triggered by a specific irregular heartbeat. However, there are times when it can be difficult to determine the reason behind that triggered heartbeat. In the case of some individuals, there is no discernible root cause. Afib is a condition that frequently runs in families, and research is continuously producing new information to help us learn more about it. Therefore, if someone in your immediate family has atrial fibrillation (Afib), you have a "family history" of the condition and, as a result, a greater likelihood of developing it yourself.

Is It Possible That Anxiety Could Cause Atrial Fibrillation?

We do not have a complete understanding of the connections between anxiety and atrial fibrillation. According to the findings of some studies, Afib can trigger anxious feelings (if you have Afib, you might worry about your symptoms or quality of life). However, only a few studies have investigated anxiety as a possible cause of atrial fibrillation. It is a well-established fact that anxiety can increase one's risk of developing cardiovascular disease and contributes to a rise in that risk that is approximately 48 percent greater. However, additional research is required to determine whether or not anxiety disorders can trigger atrial fibrillation.

CHAPTER THREE

Diagnosis

The electrical activity in your heart is the primary focus of the examination that your doctor will perform. They will most likely conduct some tests in order to figure out what is going on. The following are some of the tests that may be performed to diagnose atrial fibrillation: • Blood tests to check your thyroid, liver, and kidneys

• An electrocardiogram, also known as an EKG, to record the rate at which your heart is beating as well as the timing of the electrical signals that are traveling through it. Approximately twelve small, adhesive sensors will be placed on your chest by a nurse or technician. They are linked by wires to the apparatus that is performing the measurements.

• An x-ray of your chest to rule out the possibility that you have lung disease as the root of your issues.

• The echocardiogram, which captures a video of your heart in action through the use of sound waves

• CT scans, which are specialized X-rays that create a three-dimensional image of your heart. •

MRI scans, which use magnets and radio waves to create still images and videos of your heart. • Exercise stress tests, which evaluate how well your heart functions when you are physically active. You could walk on a treadmill or ride a stationary bike while wearing sensors that were connected to an electrocardiogram (EKG) machine. • In addition, the doctor may make use of some specialized equipment in order to learn more about the rhythm of your heart, such as the following:

• Holter monitor: It's possible that your physician will instruct you to carry around this piece of equipment with you for a few days as you go about your daily routine. It functions similarly to a portable electrocardiogram in that it continuously records data from your heart. Your doctor will be able to identify signs of an arrhythmia with its help. It's possible that you'll need a different kind of monitor for a longer period of time if your AFib symptoms come and go.

Treatment For Patients Suffering From Atrial Fibrillation (Afib)

The severity of the symptoms, as well as whether or not they have recently emerged or have been present for some time, will be taken into account by the attending physician when making the diagnosis. During the course of this evaluation, the patient might be referred to a cardiologist, who is a specialist in heart conditions. The type of atrial fibrillation, the severity of symptoms, the underlying cause, and the patient's overall health all play a role in determining the treatment option that is most appropriate. There are general guidelines available for the treatment of AFib, but the vast majority of doctors modify these guidelines in order to provide the most effective care for each patient, making treatment patient-specific. The goals of treatment for atrial fibrillation include resetting the rhythm of the heart, controlling the rate of the heart, and reducing or preventing blood clots.

Atrial fibrillation (AFib) treatment in the comfort of one's own home: is it possible?

During an active episode of atrial fibrillation, there is no effective treatment that can be done at home. If, on the other hand, the physician suggests alterations to your way of life or prescribes medication, you should carry out those recommendations to the letter. Alterations to one's way of life may be able to prevent atrial fibrillation that is associated with holiday heart. In addition, maintaining a high level of adherence to one's medication regimen while at home has the potential to prevent many instances of atrial fibrillation. This is the only way to evaluate the efficacy of the medical treatment and determine if any changes are necessary.

What are the Objectives of Medical Treatment for Atrial Fibrillation (AFib)?

Traditional treatments for atrial fibrillation focus on three primary objectives: lowering the patient's heart rate, regaining and preserving normal heart rhythm, and avoiding the formation of blood clots that could result in a stroke.

• Rate control of the heart The primary objective of the treatment is to reduce the rate of the ventricles if they are beating too quickly.

o If a patient presents with serious clinical symptoms in the emergency department, such as chest pain or shortness of breath related to the ventricular rate, the medical professional in the emergency department will make an effort to reduce the patient's heart rate as quickly as possible by administering intravenous (IV) medications.

o Patients who do not have any life-threatening symptoms may be able to take their medications orally.

o It's possible that patients will need to take more than one kind of oral medication to get their heart rate under control.

• Restore and maintain a normal cardiac rhythm: Approximately half of people who have recently been diagnosed with atrial fibrillation will return to a normal rhythm on their own within 24 to 48 hours after receiving the diagnosis. Despite this, atrial fibrillation typically reappears in a significant number of patients.

It has been established that not all people diagnosed with atrial fibrillation need to take medication in order to keep a normal heart rhythm.

o Whether or not an individual is prescribed rhythm-controlling medication, which is more commonly referred to as anti-arrhythmia medication, is partially determined by the frequency with which arrhythmia returns as well as the symptoms that it causes.

o In order to achieve the desired effect, which is a normal cardiac rhythm, medical professionals carefully customize the anti-arrhythmic medication(s) prescribed to each individual patient.

o An undesirable side effect of the majority of these medications is that they have restricted application. It is important to consult a medical professional before taking any of these medications.

• Take precautions to avoid the formation of blood clots, which can lead to strokes, which are a devastating complication of atrial fibrillation. When the atria's normal motion is disrupted, as it is in AFib, the potential exists for the formation of blood clots. A piece of a blood clot that was formed in the heart can break off and travel to the brain, where it can obstruct the flow of blood to the brain and cause a stroke.

o Preexisting medical conditions, such as high blood pressure, congestive heart failure, abnormalities of the heart valves, or coronary heart disease, significantly increase the risk of having a stroke. The risk of stroke also increases with age, particularly after the age of 65.

o To reduce their chances of having a stroke or heart failure, a significant number of people who have atrial fibrillation take the blood-thinning and anti-clotting medication known as warfarin

(Coumadin). Warfarin is able to inhibit the activity of certain factors in the blood that are responsible for clotting. Heparin administered intravenously or subcutaneously is the initial blood thinner that is used to rapidly thin a patient's blood. After that, a determination is made regarding whether or not they require oral warfarin.

o Individuals who have a lower risk of having a stroke and those who are unable to take warfarin may benefit from taking aspirin. Plavix can be taken concurrently with this medication. There are some drawbacks associated with the use of aspirin, such as increased risk of bruising and bleeding and stomach ulcers.

o Clopidogrel (Plavix) is another medication that is used to prevent the formation of clots in cardiovascular diseases such as atrial fibrillation. Numerous medical professionals use this medication.

o Other medications, such as enoxaparin (Lovenox), dabigatran (Pradaxa), and rivaroxaban, are also options for cardiologists who want to treat their patients (Xarelto). It is common for the patient's problems with

Coumadin, as well as the cardiologist's personal preference or previous experience with the drug in question, to play a role in the selection of the drugs that are used to lower the risk of blood clot formation in patients diagnosed with chronic atrial fibrillation (AFib).

What kinds of medical procedures are used to treat atrial fibrillation (also known as AFib)?

Cardioversion, also known as defibrillation or electrical cardioversion, consists of the following steps: This method involves "shocking" the heart back into its normal sinus rhythm with an electrical current in order to perform the technique. This process is also known as DC cardioversion at times. Many patients, prior to undergoing cardioversion, have a sonogram of their heart performed in order to determine whether or not any clots are present.

To perform cardioversion, a device known as an external defibrillator is attached to the chest using patches or paddles. When this procedure is carried out in a medical facility, an anesthetic is typically administered first to the patient so that they are sedated and asleep during the procedure because the electrical discharge is painful. Cardioversion is very effective; the majority of patients convert to sinus rhythm after the procedure. If the atrial fibrillation is just starting, it has the best chance of being successfully treated (that is, hours, days, or a few weeks). • Because cardioversion raises the risk of stroke and therefore typically requires pretreatment with an anticoagulant medication, it is not a permanent solution for many people because the arrhythmia frequently returns after the procedure.

Cardioversion through the use of drugs: The process of cardioversion involves the administration of anti-arrhythmic drugs either orally or intravenously in order to assist in the restoration of a normal heart rhythm. In most cases, this will take place in a hospital setting with continuous heart monitoring.

Catheter ablation, also known as radiofrequency ablation (RF ablation), is a procedure that uses radio waves to electrically burn or destroy some of the abnormal conduction pathways in the atria. This procedure is performed through a catheter.

- After threading a catheter into the atria, radiofrequency energy is delivered (in the form of heat) through the catheter to disrupt (ablate) a portion of the abnormal electrical conduction pathway. Because of this, the abnormal pathway is deactivated, which results in a flow of electrical impulses from the SA node that is more consistent. The process is also known as radiofrequency ablation in some circles.

• At this time, radiofrequency (RF) ablation is recommended for patients with atrial fibrillation who have either tried anti-arrhythmic medications without having any success or who are unable to take these medications. The most recent success rates fall somewhere between sixty and seventy percent. Before deciding to go through with this procedure, you and your doctor should have an in-depth conversation about the potentially serious complications associated with it. One of these complications is the loss of effective electrical activity in the atria, for example.

• The majority of the patient's atria's electrical activity may need to be suppressed in order to treat the patient. As a consequence of this, patients who are diagnosed with this condition need to have a pacemaker implanted (for more information on this topic, see below).

- In 2011, the Food and Drug Administration (FDA) gave its approval for the use of AtriCure, which is an ablation system, to treat atrial fibrillation in patients who were going to undergo open concomitant coronary artery bypass graft (CABG) surgery and/or valve replacement or repair.

- Cryoablation surgery is another method that can be used to treat atrial fibrillation. During this procedure, a catheter is threaded into the atrium, placed adjacent to veins that are causing abnormal atrial electrical activity, and then freezes the venous tissue to stop the activity.

Pacemaker: A pacemaker is an electronic device that prevents slow heartbeats and may reduce the likelihood of atrial fibrillation in some patients. Pacemakers are used in a relatively small percentage of patients. When the so-called "natural pacemaker," the SA node, is unable to do its job, the artificial pacemaker steps in to provide the necessary electrical impulses to keep the heart beating in a normal rhythm. • In most cases, the pacemaker is placed in both the right atrium and the right ventricle of the patient's heart. The patient's own electric impulses caused by atrial fibrillation will need to be overridden by a new atrial electrical pacemaker in order to achieve the desired results. At the moment, only a small percentage of patients are offered this procedure. This is a more complicated method and device, and there is no information about its success over the long term that is currently available. Radiofrequency ablation of the AV node, which involves disconnecting the atria from the ventricle in order to prevent rapid heart rates from being conducted to the ventricles, is sometimes performed in conjunction with the implantation of a pacemaker. • Some machines and devices in a person's environmental surroundings can interfere with the production of electrical impulses by a pacemaker. The ablation creates complete heart block, which means there is no connection between atrial electrical activity and atrial contractions and ventricular contractions. The ventricle contractions become dependent on the artificial electrical pacemaker in the right ventricle for synchronized and regular contractions between the atria and ventricles. For instance, the security measures at airports may render certain pacemakers inoperable. People need to educate themselves on the different kinds of devices that could have this impact on their pacemaker so that they can avoid using those devices. It is the responsibility of both the physician treating the patient who inserts the pacemaker and the manufacturer of the device to educate the patient on how to use the device, its limitations, and any potential complications. Patients should not be afraid to ask any questions they might have regarding the device, and those who have pacemakers should always carry an identification card that describes their condition. When going through airport security, it is possible that it will be necessary to present this identification and request that you be subject to a hand search. This is because certain security machines can deactivate pacemakers. Patients have an obligation to inform any member of the medical or dental staff that they encounter that they are wearing a pacemaker.

THE END

Made in the USA
Coppell, TX
13 September 2022